MAKE YOUR OWN WALKING PROGRAM

I0440641

WALKING CAN MAKE A HEALTHY NEW YOU

By Jessy Colter

Make Your Own Walking Program: Walking Can Make A Healthy New You

TABLE OF CONTENTS

Disclaimer

CHAPTER 1

Create Your Own Walking Program

People walk because it's easy to do. Not only is it easy, but it doesn't cost a cent to enjoy fresh air and sunshine. Plus, you gain the added bonus of experiencing new sights - depending on the area where you walk.

It's also relaxing, has the ability to relieve stress and can give you a deep sense of peace that lasts long after the walk is finished. But besides all of the fun things you can see and the stress relief you get, walking has a ton of health benefits that anyone can enjoy.

Why Walk?

Even if you walk just to get out of the house, you're going to reap some rewards for your body from this simple movement. By doing something that's easy and fun, you reward your body with a healthier, longer life.

Many health related problems are directly related to a lack of movement. The more sedentary a person is, the higher the risk they have of experiencing a serious health issue – and a shorter lifespan.

Walking is one of the easiest ways that you can prevent health problems. This simple, yet effective means of exercise is a great way to lose weight, build your muscles, add bone strength and relieve overall body tension.

Even if you don't have a family history of strokes, you'll want to do what you can to keep this health emergency at bay. Strokes are not only debilitating, but they can also lead to death.

In fact, out of all the possible causes of health related fatalities, strokes are third on the list. Yet, more than half of all strokes are preventable. A stroke happens when the flow of blood to the brain is impeded.

There are two common kinds of stroke. One is a hemorrhagic stroke and the other is an Ischemic stroke. Ischemic strokes are more likely to happen than a hemorrhagic one.

When plaque builds up in an artery, this type of stroke occurs. This plaque narrows the arteries and though this can happen as you age, you can bring on a stroke by engaging in some of the known risk behaviors.

These risk behaviors include smoking and the overuse of alcoholic beverages. But the risks are also elevated when you're overweight, when you have cholesterol numbers that are too high or when you have high blood pressure.

People who have diabetes are at greater risk than people who don't have the disease. But also on the list of risky behaviors is living a sedentary lifestyle. Even if you absolutely hate exercising, you want to do something that cuts your risk of having a stroke.

Most people choose walking because it doesn't seem like it's a form of exercise. There are a lot of ways that you can make walking something that you look forward to doing.

You can start at any age and the earlier that you start a walking program, the better your health can be. By the time you reach your mid 50s, your chance of having a stroke increases - and if you add the risky behaviors, that increase is even greater.

The aftermath of a stroke leaves behind brain cells that can be irreparably damaged. You can experience cognitive problems. This means that your memory and ability to pay attention and communicate can be affected.

You can develop aphasia, dysarthria or dyspraxia. All of these involve trouble speaking and trouble understanding speech. You may lose the ability to write and to understand what others have written.

Many people who experience a stroke can picture the words and how they want to communicate after a stroke - but the ability to make that known can be lost. Fifty percent of all stroke victims deal with depression after the event as they struggle to come to terms with the sense of what was altered or forever lost.

Some of these people struggle with personality changes or angry outbursts. Physically, there can also be a loss of limb strength or even complete use. Difficulty walking is common, as is a partial or complete loss of independence.

Incontinence is common as are eyesight problems - such as a limited ability to move the eyes or nystagmus. While you can't control the factors that you were born with that can cause health problems that lead to strokes, you can lower your odds of having one of these life-altering health issues.

With a regular walking program, you can decrease your risk of a stroke significantly over those who don't walk. Besides cutting down on your odds of having a stroke, you can improve your heart health.

In fact, your heart stands to gain quite a lot of benefits when you walk. Your heart is an organ that has a lot of responsibilities to all of the other parts of your body. It's tasked with making sure that your organs get the blood and the oxygen that they need to stay in good shape.

So if your heart suffers, so do all of the other organs in your body. Not only can the organs in your body experience trouble if your heart's not in good shape, but your muscles and joints can, too.

This is one of the reasons that you can end up with swelling around the ankles. If your heart isn't working properly, it causes fluid to accumulate. While the heart is an organ, it's muscular in nature, which means that movement such as walking strengthens the heart.

It enables it to do its job better and with less effort. Coronary diseases can be reduced or avoided in many cases when you walk regularly. You can lower your risk of developing coronary disease even if you have a family history filled with risk factors.

By engaging in a regular walking program, you can bring down your risk level to the point where it's lower than that of someone who doesn't have any coronary disease factors at all.

If you walk briskly, you can give your heart the same health benefits that you would gain if you ran on a regular basis. Medical studies presented by the American Heart Association showed that some of the benefits you gain include lower cholesterol and lower high blood pressure numbers.

You'll also have better blood flow. Your heart will have an easier time circulating the blood that your body needs to ensure proper organ function. Your organs will also gain better oxygen levels when the heart gets the exercise it needs.

Your blood pressure numbers can be improved with walking. Having high blood pressure is a risky health condition because there are often no symptoms until the pressure has been high for years.

This elevation can cause damage to your arteries. With an elevated blood pressure, your heart has to double its efforts to get the blood through your body. Untreated high blood pressure - or blood pressure that's poorly controlled - can lead to your heart becoming enlarged.

Walking keeps your blood pressure lowered, which means that the pressure of the blood flowing to and from the heart isn't as high. Regular walking can even lower your blood pressure to the point that you may be able to reduce or eliminate the amount of blood pressure medication you take.

Another heart benefit with walking is that you can also lessen your LDL cholesterol level, which is one of the main culprits in heart disease. You want to strive for this benefit because LDL cholesterol can narrow the arteries used to take blood to the heart.

This causes your body to not get the right amount of oxygen to the heart and you could end up having a heart attack. When you walk, not only can you lower the numbers on your LDL cholesterol level, but you can also raise your HDL level.

Pre-diabetes can be eliminated and diabetes sugar levels can be controlled with walking. According to the CDC, the number of people with diabetes stands at 29 million and growing.

More than 8 million people don't even know they have the disease. Not knowing and having poor control of this disease can lead to a host of severe complications - including kidney failure, limb amputation and blindness.

Pre-diabetes cases once topped a shocking 86 million cases. With most people unaware that they have it, their odds are higher of developing diabetes. Of all of the causes of death, diabetes charts the list at number seven.

Yet, it's a disease that can be avoided and can be well controlled so that it doesn't lead to an early death. Though family history does play a role in whether or not someone will get this disease, you can lower your risk factor of getting it.

One of the ways that you can do this is through walking. Walking lowers the risk factor as well as turns back the odds of pre-diabetes swinging over into full-blown diabetes.

If you already do have diabetes, then walking can help lower higher blood sugar readings. You'll also gain improvement in your blood circulation, which can help stave off blood flow complications often caused by the disease.

You gain more insulin receptors when you walk. These receptors are what the body uses to help facilitate the proper use of glucose so you end up with better sugar control.

By walking to help stave off or control diabetes, you help prevent complications to your kidneys, your heart, your eyes and your limbs. You lower your risk for stroke as well.

Your skeletal structure is strengthened when you walk. You want this strength to help you fight against fractures. Bone fractures are painful to deal with. They take several weeks to heal - and depending on the location of the fracture, they can interfere with your work or life activities.

When you walk, if you do it on a consistent basis, you can cut your risk of experiencing a bone fracture. It helps because of two reasons. First, because when you walk, you strengthen your muscles and improve your flexibility. Secondly, you gain bone density.

Some people think of bones as a part of the body that doesn't grow after a certain age. While that might be true when it comes to height, your bones are made up of living tissue.

This tissue needs exercise in order to remain strong and viable. New cells are formed, which help in the increase of density within the bones. This is especially helpful to older people who are at risk of hip fractures.

Having denser bones can stave off hip fractures. The more you walk, the better your bones will do when it comes to strength. Having stronger bones helps fight against getting a fracture in case you fall or get injured.

If you walk, even if it's only short distances, you can prevent bone density loss. This lowers your risk of developing osteoporosis. Your bones and muscles aren't the only recipients of good health when you walk.

Your brain gains from it as well. Your memory can be improved by walking. The hippocampus in the brain is positively affected and new brain cells are stimulated to grow.

As you age, your brain has some minor shrinkage. But walking helps prevent the shrinkage in the cortex that's associated with memory. This improvement in the brain is a way that can also help prevent dementia.

Walking can also be a great way to stimulate your brain. By taking along an iPod Touch or other device, you can listen to audiobooks as you walk - learn a language and more.

The more active that you keep your body, the better it is for your brain's function. The way that you feel can also be affected by your walking. Your mood can be lifted because endorphins are released when you walk.

These act as a natural mood stabilizer that can last all day, making you feel upbeat. Anxiety can be helped with a walking program and so can depression. Anger is another emotion that can affect your moods, yet can be improved with walking.

By walking when you're struggling with something emotionally, you can gain a release from the inner turmoil. And you'll be doing something healthy for your body while you're helping your mood.

If you take a survey, you'll discover that plenty of people want to have a long and healthy life. But many of these people are sabotaging that desire by being too sedentary.

The simple act of going for a walk a few times a week will add years to your life. You get these additional years because walking helps keep your organs healthy by preventing conditions such as high blood pressure, high cholesterol and various kinds of heart diseases.

You'll gain health benefits like stronger bones and better agility when you move. Studies have long shown that going for walks can help you get more restful sleep when you go to bed.

A walking program can prevent obesity or help you lose weight so that you're no longer classified as obese. While obesity can be brought on by health conditions and some medications, one of the most well known causes is overeating followed by a lack of exercise.

Not exercising causes more obesity related complications and deaths than is caused by the use of tobacco products. The CDC statistics show that over 78 million people are obese.

Obesity can lead to health conditions that are preventable with weight loss and regular exercise. The reason behind not exercising varies, depending on who you ask.

It can be because of time limitations or not wanting to join a gym or not wanting to exercise alone. Yet, walking is one of the easiest forms of exercise. You can do it at home, at the office and even on vacation.

You can use exercise equipment or walk outdoors. The possibilities are virtually endless. And unlike fancy gym memberships that require a commitment and a monthly expense, walking doesn't cost you anything - except maybe the cost of a good pair of walking shoes.

Walking is the easiest and most affordable method of improving your health, your longevity and your happiness. It's something that you can start out slowly with and build up.

Even if you hate exercising, give walking a try. You might just discover that you really like the way that walking makes you feel on a daily basis and when you implement it for more than two weeks, you'll really see a change in your life.

CHAPTER 2

Make Sure You Have the Right Equipment

Having the right equipment when you walk will make your experience the best that it can be. The main piece of equipment that you use for walking is a pair of shoes.

So you want to start your walking program by making sure that you have the right kind for your feet. Your feet aren't formed exactly like anyone else's feet are and you need to cater to the shape of your foot - especially when it comes to the arch.

This can help make a difference in giving you a pleasant walking experience as well as helping you avoid injuries. Even though a pair of shoes might claim to be good to use as walking shoes, it doesn't automatically mean that they are.

There are some specific features and details that you'll need to look for. If you're not sure how to choose the right ones, you'll want to follow these tips. One of the most common problems that people run into when they walk is the development of blisters.

Blisters develop when there's friction - something is rubbing an area of the foot. Poor fitting shoes can cause blisters and they can be caused by shoes that are either too loose or too tight.

Shoes that are too loose can rub up and down, such as against the back of the heel. Shoes that are too tight can force your toes into each other and cause pressure blisters.

Wearing the wrong kind of socks can also cause blisters to develop. You'll want to avoid wearing socks that are made of cotton. Cotton socks absorb sweat and moisture, keeping the wetness against your skin.

Choose to wear socks that are made of synthetic fabric instead. These will help keep your skin from staying wet. Something that can also help to keep your feet dry is buying shoes that are lightweight and give you good airflow around the foot.

You'll find this feature if you purchase shoes that are made from lightweight mesh. You do want to be careful that your feet aren't too dry. Dry skin is more prone to the development of blisters than moisturized skin is.

To avoid blisters, you'll want to buy running shoes that fit well, leaving the space of your finger between the end of your toes and the front of the shoe. Not only can having the right shoes help you keep blisters from forming, but it can also protect you against a common injury with your Achilles tendon.

If you've ever noticed shoes that have the notch at the back, that's what the notch is for. It's called an Achilles notch and it's located at the back center of the shoe.

It's designed that way to offer support to this tendon. You need this support when you're going to be walking short distances. Tearing your Achilles tendon can cause you to be off your feet from a couple of days to a couple of months, depending on the severity of the tear.

Something else that's an important factor to consider with the kind of walking shoes you get is the shock absorption. This is the part of the shoe that's going to be taking the brunt of the impact between your foot and whatever you're walking on.

The surface area where you're going to do your walking will greatly impact your foot's health if you don't have proper shock absorption. Walking on concrete is worse on your feet than walking on dirt or a treadmill.

The more the walking surface gives when your weight comes down on it, the less the strength of the impact. What you want to do is to pay attention to the midsole of the shoe.

This is the area at the rear or heel of the shoe that looks slightly elevated. You want the best cushioning that you can get here. The insole of the shoe is what you also want to check out before buying.

This is the part of the shoe that protects the arch of your foot. If you hold a walking shoe at eye level, you'll see the arch of the shoe. Some people add insoles for extra cushioning, but if you buy a quality shoe, you don't have to do that.

It's important that you buy shoes that are specific toward the type of arch your foot has. There are three types of arches that people have. These are average, high arch or low arch.

Low arches need shoes with more motion control. High arch feet need thicker cushioning. You can tell what kind of arch you have with your feet by wetting the bottom of your foot and stepping onto a piece of cardboard.

For people who have an average shaped arch, there will be a gently sloped indention that resembles the top center of a boomerang arch. If you have a high arch, the imprint of your foot on the cardboard will show only a very small portion of the heel.

The top of the foot imprint may even have a space between it and the bottom of the foot. Low arch feet, also known as flat feet, will show almost all of the footprint on the cardboard.

Those who have normal arches can wear whatever kind of walking shoe that they choose because their feet are better shaped to absorbed shock. High arch shaped feet need a shoe that offers great midsole cushioning, since their arch doesn't give them this necessary support.

Feet with high arches are at a higher risk of joint damage if improper shoes are worn. If you have flat feet, you need to buy walking shoes that offer stability and better midsole support.

Once you have the shoes that suit your foot style, you'll want to focus on the kind of clothing that you'll need to wear. Since your walking program is something that you'll want to stick with long term, you'll need a few days' worth of clothing to use.

It's important that you choose walking clothes that are weather appropriate. If you choose clothes that are too hot for summertime use, you can run the risk of having a heat stroke.

If you choose clothes that are too cool for winter use, you can end up chilled. Never layer up too heavily when you go for a walk in the cooler weather. Remember that whatever type of weather, you'll be walking in the body heat you'll generate from moving and will make it anywhere from 10 to 15 degrees warmer.

If it's 40 degrees outside, your body heat will make it feel like it's 50 to 55 degrees. If you layer up too much, you can be at risk of overheating - even if it's cold out.

You want the clothes that you choose to be comfortable. Clothes that don't fit right will cause chafing and you'll be miserable. It can be tempting to wear loose clothes, but loose clothes contribute to chafing.

Instead, you want clothes that fit your body snugly. Avoid cotton clothing because when you sweat, cotton will take in the moisture and this wetness contributes to chafing.

Lycra clothing is a good choice. For women, you'll want to choose a variety of sports bras that help keep you comfortable while you're walking. When these bras get stretched out, you'll need to replace them, because any sign of stretching means that the bra has lost its ability to give you the kind of support you need.

You may want to look for clothing that's similar to what runners wear. These items are made to keep the body cool and dry or warm and dry. You don't want to wear cotton clothing in any outer or innerwear since they hold on to moisture.

Wearing cotton underwear can cause chafing in the inner creases of the groin where it meets the leg. You also want to avoid clothing with inside material that can pull.

These kinds of materials, such as some styles of sweatpants, can cause chafing. If you want the best walking clothes, you're going to want to shop for flexible fabrics.

These are clothing items that are made of lightweight material and have some give to them despite being fitted. These kinds of materials allow for more natural movements as you walk.

Walking is one of the safest ways to get moving, but it's not without its need to take some precautions. One of the precautions that you're going to want to take is to protect yourself against damage from the sun.

Sun damage is one of the most overlooked injuries when it comes to walking. Most people simply don't think about protecting their skin since they're just going to be out for a little while.

But you want to use sunscreen regardless of how long you plan to be on your walk. The purpose of sunscreen is to keep the sun's harmful rays from causing damage such as wrinkles and sunspots, and also cell changes that could cause skin cancer to develop.

Even on overcast days, your skin can be at risk. You'll want to check what your day's UV rating or index is before venturing out. Some smart technology devices have apps that will give you the UV index in your area.

The lower the number given, the less risk you are to overexposure to the sun's rays. If you're going to be out walking in hot weather, it's possible that you'll sweat off the sunscreen that you applied at the beginning of the walk.

The brand that you choose to use may suggest that you reapply it after a certain amount of time. Not only is your skin subject to damage from the sun's rays, but so are your eyes.

Sun damage has been linked with certain eye problems. It's best to wear sunglasses on bright sunny days to avoid damage to your eyes. Some walkers choose to wear sun visors to add protection against ultraviolet rays.

Sunscreen that contains an SPF level of 15 is a good choice for most walkers. However, if you're someone who's had a problem with skin cancer in the past or you're at higher risk because of family genetics, then you'll want to use one with an SPF level of 30 or higher.

Make sure that you check the ingredients list. Not all sunscreens are the same - and some have less effective ingredients than others. You'll also want to check the expiration date of a sunscreen before you use it.

Some can lose their effectiveness sooner than other brands can. When applying sunscreen, make sure that you don't forget about the top of your head. Scalp sunburns can be painful and the scalp is one of the most often overlooked places when applying sunscreen.

When starting a walking program, some people like to walk outdoors very early in the morning, while others like to walk later in the evening. This is especially true when the weather is too hot to be comfortable in the middle of the day.

While this might make you more comfortable, it also raises the risk factor that you could end up with an injury or have your safety compromised in other ways. This is why you'll want to buy safety gear for your walking program.

You'll want to buy items such as reflective gear. When you're wearing reflective gear, it makes it easier for you to be seen. By being more visible, you can cut your risk of ending up getting hurt by traffic because a driver didn't see you in the early morning or evening darkness.

Plus, if you happen to fall or are unable to continue walking, reflective gear can make it easier for other people to be able to locate you. Most of the reflective gear that you can get are lightweight and easy to make a part of your walking routine.

You can get vests designed to fit men or women. These vests fit right over your walking clothes. They have wide stripes that reflect light and make you clearly visible to others walking or to oncoming traffic.

Ankle bands are another type of reflective gear that can make you more noticeable as you walk. Flashing armbands and personal safety lights can alert others to your presence in an area.

Even if you don't plan to walk when it's dark out, it's always a good idea to have this gear. Many walkers have started out on their planned location only to find themselves out later than they intended.

They end up walking home in the dark. LED wrist lights can also be helpful as safety gear for walkers. If you live in an area that's known for higher temperatures in the summer, you might want to think about making sure you stay hydrated during your walk.

You can do this by taking water with you. If you don't want to carry the water, you can bring it along by using a hydration belt or an armband water carrier. Walking is a great way to clear your head and get some much needed mental relaxation.

If you're going to be walking outside, you can take along a portable entertainment device such as an iPod Touch. With one of these, you can listen to your favorite music.

You can hear an audiobook or you can take in the talk show that you enjoy. You can also enjoy entertainment apps on your iPhone. You can learn a new language, catch up on sports or talk with friends.

Sometimes, you'll find that you can't follow your outdoor walking program like you want to do and you may end up having to rely on your treadmill. Boredom while walking on a treadmill is one of the reasons that it's favored less than walking outdoors.

But you can beat boredom by choosing a treadmill that helps you be entertained while you're walking. You can get treadmills that have desk stands so you can use your laptop, watch television, listen to music or learn educational material.

CHAPTER 3
Mapping Out the Location of Your Walking Regimen

Finding a place to walk isn't difficult, but you do want to plan ahead. If you have areas near your home where you can walk, these can be convenient. And studies have shown that the more convenient and more accessible a walking area is, the more likely it will be that you'll stick with a walking program.

This means that if you can, you should seek to find an area that you can access right out of your front door. If you live in a suburban neighborhood, you'll likely have sidewalks or walking trails where you can plan your course.

You can measure off the distance that you walk by driving your car the length of your route. Or you can figure it up by using a pedometer Taking around 2,000 steps equals one mile.

Walking outdoors in your neighborhood can be a great way to get involved with people who are also walking in the area. Plus, it's a good way to meet and get to know the people in your neighborhood.

You might even be able to find a walking partner this way if you want one. Statistics show that a person who lives in a neighborhood that has walking areas gets more exercise, more fresh air and loses an average of 10 pounds more than people who live in neighborhoods without walking areas.

There are sites online that will give a neighborhood a score based on how walkable the area is. Some neighborhoods are more walker friendly than others. You can tell if your neighborhood is good to walk in by seeing if it meets the following criteria:

First, there should be plenty of room to walk. The areas or sidewalks should be wide and roomy enough so that two people can pass side by side when approaching from opposite sides.

The sidewalks or walking areas should be smooth and free of trash and other debris.

There should be well marked lines if you have to cross the street. If you have to go across a road that's busy with a steady flow of traffic, there should be designated crosswalks, stop signs or pedestrian signals.

Walking safely should be a priority - and if you have to take risks to walk in your neighborhood, then it's better to find another designated walk area.

Walking trails and sidewalks are considered to be one of the safer ways to walk outdoors. But, even if you live in a more rural area, you can still find a decent place to walk not far from your home.

As long as you walk with the traffic, you can walk along the side of the roads. But if you're in an area that's fairly isolated, you might want to walk with a partner for safety reasons.

You also want to make sure that you're visible if you're walking during the twilight or evening hours. Some people choose to incorporate their walking program with the time they spend making sure their dogs get adequate exercise.

So tying the two of these together would also be a great motivator to stick with a program. Not everyone lives in a neighborhood that's walker friendly, but that doesn't mean that you still can't meet your walking goals.

In most of the states, there are what's known as walking hot spots. These are places that are well known that many people choose to use to keep up their walking program.

You may not be aware of them, but they're easy to find. For a designated local hot spot for walking in your area, you can do a search online to see the ones that are near you.

The American Heart Association has a list of walking paths. All you have to do is type in a search engine box the words organization plus walking paths. A list of what's available will pop up.

These walking areas are broken down by states where they're found as well as whether the path is easy or difficult. This is a good way to keep up your walking if you go on vacation, too.

You can look in advance for walking areas in the state that you're going to be traveling to. By searching online, you'll also find walking clubs and an online walking tracker so that you can view your progress at a glance.

You want to find an area that you enjoy walking in and it can help if you're just starting a walking program if you have some support for what you want to do. There are walking chapters in various states and some have several.

You can go online, type in the state that you live in and search for "walking chapters." Not only will you get several choices in some cases, but you'll also find guidance on how to start one if there's not one in your area but you'd like there to be.

There are walking clubs for many different interests and compatibility levels. You can find walking clubs for seniors or ones for men or women. You'll find clubs for young moms that meet when the kids are in school.

You'll find ones that meet with families that have young children and parents bring a stroller along for the walks. You'll find walking clubs where pets are also part of the walking program.

Whatever your interests are, you're sure to find a walking club that's a match for you. You can also find walking events that promote walking in conjunction with a good cause - such as raising awareness for a health issue or for a non-profit organization.

Some of these event attendees meet on a regular basis to walk. If there's an association that promotes awareness about a disease, you can check with those for walking programs as well.

For example, if you check with the American Diabetes Association, you'll see that they offer some helpful tips about walking and walking programs. You can join a team of walkers or start a team.

There are events that are kid friendly walking programs that are held to promote families walking together. You can find these listed on your community's website page or by contacting your local community center.

Promoting walking programs and using specifically designated areas is something that many hospitals support. You can find these by searching through their health and wellness programs.

Some schools also have community involved events where walking programs are offered as a way to encourage students to be healthier. You'll find these in schools from elementary all the way to college level.

There are some corporations that offer walking programs under workplace wellness programs or employee wellness programs. Many of these corporations also offer discounted group membership if employees who are part of the walking program also want to join a weight loss program as a group.

There are medical insurance companies that reward members who take part in walking programs and other healthy activities by offering them lowered premiums.

A few companies offer extra perks like points that can be earned toward gift card redemption. Walking outdoors alone, with a partner, or as part of a group, can be fun - a way to get healthier and to lose any extra pounds you want to take off.

But unfortunately, the weather doesn't always like to play along. While walking in a light drizzle might not be too bad, when it's a torrential downpour outside, walking can be pretty miserable and it can be easy to let the motivation slide.

Especially if you encounter several days where the weather is just too bad to be out walking in it. For that reason, you need to have a backup plan. By having a backup plan, you can keep your motivation strong.

It's easier to break a habit than it is to keep it up. By having a contingency plan, you won't lose the steam you've already built up. One of the great ways that you can get your steps in if the weather won't allow you to do it walking outdoors is by walking indoors at your local shopping mall.

Most malls will allow walkers to use their space specifically for walking. There are several walking groups that have permission to walk in malls all across America. If that sounds like something that you'd like, you can call the local mall in your area and ask about it.

If you don't want to go walking at the mall alone, you can do a search for mall walkers in your area and you'll find groups that you can meet up with. Plus, you can develop some lasting friendships while you're sticking with your walking program.

Sometimes the days just won't line up for you to make it out to the mall or any other place where you would normally walk. You may not feel like getting out of the house that day.

Or maybe going out to the mall to walk when the weather is bad is just not something that you enjoy doing. Sometimes the weather just isn't safe to be out and about in - like if the roads are icy.

You won't want to risk falling and injuring yourself or having your vehicle slide on a patch of ice to get anywhere. For that reason, you want to make sure that you have a way to get your walking in at home so that you can continue to reach your walking program goals.

With that in mind, you'll want to use a treadmill. If you don't have one yet, you can find a variety of great treadmills for reasonable costs and many of these will fold up out of the way for maximum space saving perks.

One of the biggest reasons that people don't really like to use a treadmill as part of a walking routine is that using a treadmill doesn't off the same sense of stimulation that being outdoors offers.

It also doesn't give a person the same sensory stimulation as walking at the mall. The best way to use a treadmill is by not walking on it for a continual amount of time.

It's best to use a treadmill if you break up the time you're walking on it. You can create intervals that give you the same amount of benefit that you'd find by continual walking outdoors.

If you normally walk for half an hour each time you go out, you'll want to divide your treadmill time by three 10 minute walks or six 5 minute walks. You need to make sure that you keep your motivation up.

So what you can do is to give yourself a mini goal. Aim for to cover a certain amount of distance in your first time on the treadmill. When you get back on after the first interval, push yourself to beat your first time.

By giving yourself different kinds of mini challenges, you'll stave off boredom and keep yourself motivated. You can also change the incline of the treadmill so that you're walking at an uphill angle.

Some people will use a treadmill for their walking program and walk while watching a nature video. These are videos that mimic a walk outside. You can find ones that show a walk through a forest.

On the video, you'll see blue skies, thick trees and even hear birds chirping along as you walk. Or, you can find videos that will mimic taking a walk along a tropical road by the water.

In the video, you'll see palm trees waving and hear the breeze blowing gently. Using a nature video while walking on a treadmill is a good way to keep you from feeling like you're cooped up inside.

When you're just starting out with something, it can seem like it's a lot of fun and excitement. But when you fall into a rut of doing the same thing at the same time every week, eventually, the fun level will diminish.

Regardless of your favorite location for your walking program, it's always best to have as many choices as possible. This is one of the best ways that you can make sure that you don't encounter boredom.

Getting bored when it comes to any kind of exercise, low intensity, moderate, or high activity is something that's normal. Everyone will experience some form of boredom at one point or another.

However, boredom is one of the biggest drawbacks to sticking with any kind of walking program. When something becomes boring, it seems like getting it done is more of a chore.

If this starts with you, then you'll discover that you dread even thinking about walking and you'll find yourself starting to look for excuses to avoid it. Even doing things around the house that you hate to do will look good in comparison.

Keeping boredom at bay is one of your best offenses when it comes to sticking with a walking program because no matter how young or old you are, being bored is no fun.

There is a solution, though. If you switch up how you walk, then you end up with something new to look forward to. If you're walking in your neighborhood, what you can do is branch out and move to walking in nearby neighborhoods.

That way, you're adding steps to your daily count, seeing new sites and meeting new people on your way. When the weather's bad, if you're someone who likes to walk at the mall, you can check out a different mall but still within driving distance.

Seeing new stores with new displays can help beat boredom. You can also change up the style in which you walk. You can add a brisker pace, move your arms differently and more.

Having someone walk with you can also help beat boredom. Conversations can enrich a walk and it's always different each time that you do it. If you're walking as part of a group or organization, you can schedule to walk with different people from the group.

You might even try a walking DVD where you march in place and get inspired by the person leading the exercise. There's never a reason why walking can't be relaxing and fun.

CHAPTER 4

Setting the Perfect Pace for Your Walking Program

When you see someone zipping around a walking trail at the park, it can be easy to look at their form and how fast they're making tracks and feel envious. It can be tempting to want to copy that same pace.

But looking at where someone else is with their walking isn't something that you should do. You don't want to compare your point to someone else's because they may have been doing this a lot longer.

They might be at a different health level. All you can do is do the best that you can for you regardless of where anyone else is at in their journey. Because walking is so easy to do, it doesn't appear as if there's any special planning that needs to go into it with pacing.

You can just walk until you're tired is how most people view it. While it can be tempting to really push yourself, thinking that since it's good for you, you might as well do a lot of it quickly, watch out for this pitfall.

Walking is something that you don't want to overdo. You don't want to overdo it because it really is one of the easiest ways to get your heart pumping, gain energy, lose weight and get rid of stress.

It can also help you gain some muscle tone. Overdoing a walking program means that you're pushing your body beyond its ability to handle the physical stress.

Not slowing down when your body is giving off signals to pull back is a common factor in injuries. The best way to handle pace if you're just now beginning a walking program is to focus on long term goals and build toward those goals slowly.

This might mean that when you begin, you'll only head out for a ten minute walk and then you'll come back to your home. You'll want to build up stamina and pacing.

So what you can do is to walk for only ten minutes the first several days. Then after that, you can slowly add time increments in counts of five or ten. This way, you're building up tolerance for the walking and your muscles aren't being tasked with going all out at once.

Also, if you're the type of person who's had a fairly sedentary lifestyle, starting a walking program is going to offer some challenges with the way that you handle pacing.

It will be easier for someone who isn't used to walking to be excited about it in the beginning and end up hating it because a pace that was too fast and too long was attempted.

Even if you've been walking for awhile, if you jump in too quickly, you can overdo it and end up injuring yourself. When an injury sidelines you, it can be difficult to get your motivation back and you'll end up dealing with frustration.

Sometimes getting sidelined with an injury causes people to quit a walking program completely and you want to avoid that happening. A good rule of thumb to pay attention to when you're walking is how the pace makes you feel physically.

Your heart should be pumping faster, but you shouldn't feel like you're having to gasp for breath. Once you've been walking long enough so that you're comfortable with it and it's become a habit for you, you'll want to check to see how it's challenging your body.

If the pacing you're now at seems easy to you, it might be time to kick it up a notch and increase your pace. Like any form of movement, your body will let you know when you're pushing it too hard.

If you get warning signs, such as painful shins, listen to your body. Any time you have pain in your shins, it means that you're walking too fast and too far. Back off of your pacing for a few days, take it slower and let your body heal and adjust.

Many people aren't sure exactly how to set pacing when walking. The best way that you can set a healthy pace is to time yourself getting to a mile. To get to a mile, it should take a beginner about 20 minutes.

Someone who's used to walking already, can usually hit a mile at a comfortable pace within 15 minutes. Reaching a mile with a certain pacing goal will depend on how fit that you are, the way that you walk and what kind of an area you're walking in.

You'll reach your mile goal faster if you're walking on solid ground such as asphalt or a sidewalk. But walking on rough ground will slow your progress. You can judge your pacing by seeing if your heart is beating within the rate that you've targeted.

While you're walking, you should be able to speak comfortably. If you can't, then your pacing is too fast. But if you have the lung capacity to belt out your favorite fast song, then your pacing is too slow for you to really be getting much benefit from it.

You can chart your pacing by keeping a personal tracker. Write down how fast it takes you to get from one point to another at the beginning of each month. Your pacing should gradually improve from month go month.

So at the beginning of one month, if it takes you 25 minutes to get in a mile distance, by gradually increasing your pacing, you should be able to bring that down to an average of 15 minutes for a mile.

While paying attention to pacing, the way that you move your body is an important part of a walking program. You need to have good posture as you're walking to keep from injuring yourself.

Like most movements, there's a right way and a wrong way to do it. It's imperative that you use the correct form when you're walking. And by using the correct form, you'll burn a greater amount of calories.

Plus, your chances of injuring yourself will be less. You should keep your posture during a walking program in the same manner that you would normally walk as you go about your day.

When you walk, keep your head up. If you walk while looking down, this can put strain on your neck muscles. Not to mention if you're looking down while you're walking, it can make it easier to run into something in front of you.

Your chin should be straight and your shoulders relaxed. As you walk, don't lean forward. This can be a bad habit to get into. If you walk while leaning forward, you put a great amount of strain on your lower back muscles.

You can do a lot for your core muscles by walking with your stomach slightly tightened. Keep your arms bent, but not tensed. When your foot hits the ground, it should be with the heel landing first, then the toe.

Keeping up with your stride can help you get the most from a walking program. You might hear a lot of talk about stride and how many steps that it will take you to reach a mile.

But you shouldn't believe everything you hear like it's a one size fits all concept because walking for one person is not the same for another. A lot of people use this kind of advice when they're using a pedometer to measure steps.

But what you have to take into consideration is that not everyone will have the same kind of steps. Sometimes one person's stride will be a length of two or two and a half feet.

Another person's might be a stride that's longer or shorter than that. Your walking stride will depend on your gender, how you normally walk, your current physical condition and the area where you're walking.

A rougher terrain will cause you to walk at a slower stride. A brisk stride regardless of the length of the step you take is the best way to walk. You can determine how fast your stride is by how many steps that you take per minute.

Taking 100 steps a minute is considered to be a moderate walking stride. The more steps that you take per minute determines your speed. If you're new to walking, you'll want to start at a slower pace.

Aim for 50 steps per minute and gradually increase the amount. If you feel pain while you're walking, such as a stitch in your side, then you need to slow your pace.

You should keep your arms bent while you walk, but not still. Allow your arms to move back and forth in rhythm with the back and forth of your leg movements. Keep in mind that a stiff posture when walking will equal stiff muscles when you're finished with your walk.

There are some who like to add a little extra equipment to their walking program. This extra equipment is in the form of wrist or ankle weights. You will find many fitness sites that will advocate the use of these additional weights when walking.

But you should know that this really boils down to a personal choice. Walking with the use of any type of weight materials is better suited to muscle building or resistance routines.

And if you're new to a walking program, you'll want to avoid using weights - at least until you think your body is ready to level up. Listen to your body. It can advise you better than anyone else.

CHAPTER 5

Developing a Plan of Goals

There's never anything wrong with dreaming big in any area of your life. However, no big dreams are ever reached unless smaller goals are put into place.

These small goals add up to reaching the bigger goal. Plus, when you break down your larger or long term goals into smaller ones, you achieve a "can do" mindset.

This is one of the ways that helps people achieve what some see as impossible dreams. For example, if you dream of taking part in a walking event that's 15 miles long, you can certainly have that dream.

But you wouldn't leave your house and walk 15 miles if you've never walked that distance before. Instead, you would break that 15 miles down by 3 or by 5 and you would gradually build up to it.

To go all out and attempt to walk 15 miles when you've never walked more than 2 is setting yourself up for possible injury and disappointment. This is one of the reasons that so many people set resolutions - which are really just goals by another name - and then don't meet those resolutions.

They set the goal too big and too broad. Goals need to be broken down and easily defined so that they can be easily attainable. If you set a goal to walk 60 miles in a week, you'd have to walk just over 8.5 miles a day every day to reach that goal.

If you're someone who's currently walking 40 miles a week, then that goal would probably be within your reach. But for someone who's currently walking just 2 miles for the entire week, that goal would be more difficult for you to reach.

Don't let your excitement over a walking program push you to over the edge of a goal that's reasonable for you to achieve. Think progressive instead of aggressive.

Aggressive goals are usually full of zeal and run on emotion versus planning. Look out for things that can sabotage your goal. These are things that you have to take into account that must be handled as you attempt your goal.

For example, if you plan to walk 6 miles every day without fail, but you have child care issues, that can throw off your time. Your goal should be something that's concrete and easy for you to state.

The more specific a goal is, the better it is. You should be able to state in your goal why you want to walk. Some people write down that they want to get healthy.

Others choose to write down weight loss or because they want to prevent possible health problems for the future. But vague goals don't help you be specific about why you're on a walking program.

Instead of saying that you want to lose weight (if that's your goal), write down instead that you want to lose 2 pounds a week. Or that you want to lose 20 pounds by losing 2 pounds a week.

Remember to set small goals that contribute to a larger one. This way, each time that you achieve one of your smaller goals, it helps motivate you to continue striving toward your long term goal.

A goal should also be something that you can measure. When you're able to measure how you're doing on your walking program, this can help pull you back if you start to slack off.

A goal with a measure can involve time or distance, such as being able to walk 10 miles in a week within four months of beginning a walking program. Your goal should be something that's within your reach.

If you set a goal that's impossible to reach because of extenuating circumstances, it will discourage you. For example, you might be someone who struggles with health problems that makes it difficult to lose weight as fast you'd like.

If this is something you have an issue with, then you want to be careful setting time limits on how fast you want to lose weight with your walking program. A walking program is a good way to lose weight, but it needs to have goals that work for you.

It might take you longer to reach your goals if you have a greater struggle than others, but that doesn't matter if you set goals that are right for you. You do want to set due dates on your goals.

This gives you a length of time that you can aim for to accomplish it. Otherwise, it's too easy to shrug off the goal and fall into the mindset that you can try again tomorrow.

By having due dates for your goals, it helps keep pushing you forward. To get started, decide your overall goal and then break it down. Take a chart and decide where you want to be as your final goal.

If that's to walk a certain number of miles in a year, then you know you need to break down that goal by monthly goals, and then further break it down by weekly, then daily goals.

You can create a calendar where you mark down each day's steps. This will help you because you'll have a visual reminder of the progress that you've already made.

So when motivation lags, and this does happen to everyone, you'll be able to use how far you've come to push yourself to keep on going. It will be helpful for you to see that at the beginning of the month, you started out with 2,000 steps - but by the end of the month, you're already up to 5,000.

This can be especially helpful if one of your goals during your program is weight loss and you don't feel as if anything is changing. This lets you see the positive steps you're making before you'll necessarily see any changes in your body.

What some people do is base a walking program on the number of steps that they take every day. This is a great way of achieving a long term goal, but it should still be broken down into smaller goals.

The more steps that you take every day, the greater the benefit that you'll gain from that. But what most people do is aim for a certain number of steps without actually knowing the best way to reach that goal.

They try to up their step level in a day or two. There's a better way. You need to start by figuring out the number of steps that you currently walk. You can do this by wearing a pedometer for 3 to 5 days.

At the end of your determined usage, you'll have the total number of steps that you average. Once you have that, divide by the number of days that you recorded the steps.

This will give you the actual amount of steps you take a day. This number is going to vary. Some days, you might walk 3,000 steps. Other days, you might walk 5,000 steps.

The key is to use the average amount that you walk per week and increase your percentage to get your 10,000 step per day goal. It may take you a few weeks to reach that count, but you can do it by slowly adding 20% to 30% increases each day.

So if you were walking 2,500 steps a day, add 500 steps if you're using 20% increases. When you add the 500 steps, you'll be at 3,000 steps. By adding 20% to that, you'll have an additional 600 steps - or 100 more than the 500 you just added.

CHAPTER 6
Technology That Caters to Walkers

There are tools that can help you with your walking program. Some of these tools can track your steps to help you reach your goals. One of the most popular tools for walkers is a Fitbit.

This is a pedometer that takes advantage of the newest technology available to help you stay fit and healthy. It's a wonderful gadget that can be used to improve many areas of your life.

Wearable technology comes in many formats and style and has made tracking the amount of steps you take easier than ever. This can be a great motivator to use with a walking program.

One of the most popular gadgets for walkers is the Fitbit Flex Wireless Activity and Sleep Wristband. All you have to do is snap the device on your wrist like you would a watch then go about your normal activities.

Fitbit will count each step you take throughout the day whether you're walking, jogging, dancing, cleaning the house or working around the office. The device has the ability to track the distances that you've walked and how many calories you've burned with your activities.

The gadget keeps a record of how often you're active and will log your daily statistics. If you have a goal set that you want to meet with the amount of steps that you take, the Fitbit can let you know if you're on track to reach your day's step goal.

It also has the ability to send you a wakeup alarm to help you get up and get started moving. Fitbit gives users several tools that can help you stay motivated. Using the Fitbit website, you can create an account that lets you monitor your health and fitness levels.

You can log into the site, which will let you set up a personalized account. Using this personalized account, you can set goals. Remember to set ones that are reasonable for you.

Once you've set up your goal, you'll be able to see if you're reaching it by glancing at your Fitbit. This wearable pedometer has five lights. The first one lights up when you reach 20% of your goal.

The next one will light up when you've reached 40% of your goal then 60% and 80%. When the fifth light has lit, you'll know that you've reached your goal for the day.

Another great feature of the Fitbit is that you can sync wirelessly with your favorite Android or iOS device. This means that you can access your Fitbit account on your iPad, Samsung Galaxy, or iPhone.

The Fitbit app is free and works well with other fitness apps like SparkPeople and MyFitnessPal. The Fitbit is waterproof and this can be helpful if you plan on wearing it all day.

You can use your Fitbit in the shower or while swimming and not have to worry about damaging it by getting it waterlogged. You can also use your FitBit account to monitor your weight, log the foods you eat, and share your goals with your friends and family.

This is a great features because sharing your walking goals with your online community can actually help motivate you to stick to your walking program. When you reach an important milestone - like meeting your daily walking goal - Fitbit will reward you with a badge. These badges offer visual proof of your success and seeing them can drive you to accomplish your walking goals.

If you'd rather not count the steps you take during the day, you can use Fitbit to count the amount of calories burned each day or the number of minutes you've been active.

This is especially helpful if you're using your new walking program to help you lose weight. The FitBit, like most wearable technology, does have a battery that will need to be recharged.

However, each charge should allow you to use your Fitbit for 5-7 days before you have to recharge. The Fitbit is a great pedometer with some advanced features. But it's not the only gadget that counts your steps.

You should also check out the UP24 by Jawbone. The UP24 works in a similar way to the Fitbit in that it measures your steps as well as your health and fitness level.

Unlike the Fitbit, you can't change out the wristband on the UP24. This means that you have to stick with the color you originally chose. This isn't a big deal to some consumers, but others find this annoying.

While the UP24 looks similar to the Fitbit, it is chunkier. The clasp is easier to work with and you can adjust the wristband easily if needed. It weighs less than an ounce - so despite the bulky look, you won't feel like your wrist is weighed down.

The UP24 also has an app available that tracks your calories, the number of steps you've taken, and how active you've been today. The application can be used on both iOS and Android devices.

This means that you can use the app on devices like the iPhone, iPad, Samsung tablet, and more. The UP24 uses Bluetooth technology to sync your activity level with your account.

Like the Fitbit, the UP24 application is a helpful system that can give you an accurate measurement of how active you truly are. It will also help you figure out if you're not nearly as active as you thought you were.

One of the features that a lot of users like is that you can use the app to record what you're eating. It has an extremely convenient way of doing this. If you don't want to enter in your food manually, just grab a picture of the barcode.

The UP24 application can scan the barcode and will log what you've eaten. One feature that many consumers like about the UP24 is that it has an inactivity alert. If you've been inactive for a long time, the UP24 will gently vibrate against your wrist to remind you to get up and move.

This can be helpful if you spend long hours working in a sedentary job. You can set the inactivity alert on your account so that you can customize how often the alert goes out.

You could use it to remind you to take a short walk every hour or every few hours. The choice is up to you. If you want to challenge yourself, you can share your walking and fitness goals through the app.

This way, your friends and family can encourage and challenge you to meet your goals every week. The UP24 is described as water resistant. This means that you can get liquid on the device like sweat or water.

But you shouldn't submerge the UP24 under water, so make sure you remove it before swimming or other aquatic activities. The UP24 application can log and store your data for nine months.

This allows you to track your health over the course of several months. You'll be able to see what habits helped you the most and which ones didn't. Pedometers by Omron are also helpful tools for walkers.

The HJ-112 Pocket Pedometer by Omron is a good one. It has the ability to reset itself every day so that you don't have to manually subtract one day's step count from the following day.

It can hold a week's worth of information at a time. The pedometer can keep track of your step count, how long you walked, the distance that you covered and the calories that you've used.

What a lot of walkers like about this pedometer is that it can divide the amount of regular walking steps that you take from the specific brisk ones. This means that you'll be able to keep a track of just your walking program steps if you want to.

Other technology that can be helpful for walkers focuses on entertainment and motivation value. The best technology for this is music device. Having an iPod or other music device along can offer great boredom buster benefits to walkers.

One of the ways that it can help is by giving you motivation. You can use your playlist to create a walking challenge. For example, you can keep your focus on a point in the distance and aim for that point before the end of a song.

When you're starting out on your walk, you can have the slower paced songs in your playlist set to start playing. These can be your warm up songs. Then, after you've warmed up, you can switch to a moderate tempo song, followed by a song that has a fast beat.

You can use how fast or slow a song is to help you know when to change your pacing. Or, you can use a playlist to determine the journey of your walk. Music devices are great ways to set up interval walking during your time.

So if you want to walk quicker for some minutes over others, a song can help you keep track of that. Music can help shake up how you figure your accomplishments, too.

Rather than counting off the length of time you've been walking for that day, you can set it up by songs. For instance, you're going to listen to four songs that are at least four minutes long on the walk that you take for the day.

When you want to add steps to your walking routine, you can simply increase the length of your playlist and add more songs. Your walks will be a lot more enjoyable and you'll get to hear some great tunes.

If you do walk with a music device, you want to be careful that you exercise caution with the volume control. Always make sure that you can be aware of your surroundings by hearing what's going on around you.

CHAPTER 7
Problem Areas to Watch for as a Walker

Though walking is safe and easy, repeated movements can strain your muscles and joints if you're not careful. You should keep in mind that if you're feeling pain anywhere in your body while you're on a walking program, the safest bet is to see a doctor to make sure there's nothing serious going on.

Making sure a new ache or pain isn't anything serious is something that will help you keep up your momentum. Walking when you're feeling pain can cause you to change your gait to accommodate for the pain, can give you lower back aches and further damage an area that's injured – all of which can derail your walking program.

One of the ways that you can injure your knees while walking is by setting a pace that's too fast for your current fitness level. Your knees can become injured doing repetitive movement and this can cause an inflammation to build up.

You can also develop problems with your knees if you have poor posture while you're walking. One of the most common causes of knee problems usually occurs because of leaning forward or tilting back slightly as you walk.

Your joint starts to feel pressure pain - at first, you may not recognize this as joint pain. You'll only recognize that the pain seems to come from beneath your kneecap.

Then you may notice swelling or the skin in the area feels hot to the touch. This is a sign of inflammation and it needs to be treated. Sometimes simply resting the affected area can help.

You simply have to try to not use the knee as much as possible. If resting it doesn't help, then you'll need to take medication or possibly use compression bandages or a brace.

Remember that if any pain persists after home rest and treatment - get it checked. Your muscles and joints need to gradually grow accustomed to your walking program.

If you do too much too fast, that's another way that you can also hurt your knees.

Setting your walking program to cover rough terrain is also a way that your knees can be injured.

Rough terrain or areas that are at an incline can put even more pressure on the knees. The IT band is a ligament that enables you to move your knee. The ligament also helps keep it steady.

If this ligament becomes inflamed, it can make it hard for you to use the knee for any movement. This type of injury is caused by pushing yourself to walk distances that your body isn't ready to handle.

But wearing shoes that should have been replaced due to wear and tear can also cause it. Ice and rest can help alleviate the pain caused by injury to the IT band. A common injury in walkers is plantar fasciitis.

This is a condition that can cause pain that you'll feel on the bottom of one or both feet. The culprits behind this pain are tiny tears caused by overuse - such as too much walking or buying poorly cushioned shoes.

If the problem persists and you don't get it treated, then you can develop bone spurs - a condition that's even more painful. If you have feet that don't have good arches, your chance of developing a bunion is higher than that of walkers with high arches.

To avoid this condition, you need to make sure that your shoes don't fit so snugly that they press against the toe joints. Shin splints are common for walkers, too. These are bone pains that occur in the lower legs.

The pain is caused by inflammation. The inflammation is caused by doing too much walking. It's also caused by walking on terrain that has little or no give - such as asphalt.

If you continually walk briskly up or down a hill, this can contribute to shin splints. Unfortunately, some people attribute the pain from shin splints to muscle pain and try to keep on walking.

If you feel any pain in your lower leg bones, be on the safe side and suspect that the pain is from a shin splint. With this kind of injury, you should stop walking immediately.

They're a sign that damage has occurred and if you continue walking with a shin splint, you can do serious damage to the tissue and bone. If you continue to keep walking with shin splints, you'll develop serious bone fractures and this painful consequence will keep you off your feet for weeks.

Some health conditions do contribute to the development of shin splints. Among these conditions is osteoporosis. Any health condition that affects bone density can make you more susceptible to shin splints.

Because swelling occurs with shin splints, the treatment - if you happen to get this condition - is to rest the affected leg and use ice to reduce the swelling. Your leg will heal faster if you stay off of it.

You can take precautions that can help prevent you from getting shin splints. Always make sure that you're wearing the right shoes every time you go out walking.

Make sure that your shoes are in good shape and there are no worn places. Check your shoes to make sure that they're giving you the right kind of absorption protection.

Shoes that have low quality insoles don't give your legs the kind of protection that they need. It's the impact of the foot coming in contact with a surface that can lead to shin splints.

Choose to walk on areas that have more give than the asphalt. Stay away from areas that force you to flex your foot upward. If you've had a shin splint in the past, make sure that when you are able to get back to walking that you slowly build back up to the level you were at before you were injured.

If you try to jump back to where you were, you can risk a re-injury. Bursitis is an inflammation caused by walking. It happens when the fluid sac or bursae get irritated.

One of the biggest causes for hip pain from this condition is not taking the time to slowly level up to the miles you cover while walking. By taking your time to build your walking program, you can avoid many of the joint problems, injuries and inflammations that others experience.

Hamstring injuries can occur with walking if you push yourself to walk too fast - especially if you're going up inclines or hills. Your hamstring is made up of three muscles and these muscles are what allow you to bend your knee.

If you strain or pull a hamstring, it means that the muscle has torn and it could be one of any of the three muscles within the hamstring. When an injury like this occurs, you can experience muscle weakness - such as the inability to walk - as well as pain and swelling.

To avoid this kind of injury, build up your walking endurance and avoid terrain that cause for strenuous use of the hamstring muscles. Sprains are common with walking, but are easily one of the most avoidable injuries.

The two most easily sprained areas when walking are the ankles and the wrists from catching yourself if you trip and fall. With the ankles, it's easy to turn your foot and sprain it if you're walking on uneven surfaces.

Even if the surface is relatively flat - such as a road or sidewalk - there can still be small items - such as a rock or a twig - that can cause you to sprain your ankle.

Your Achilles tendon can be injured if you overuse it by walking more than you should before you're ready. To protect against injuring this tendon, you want to be careful with uphill walking or any walking that causes this muscle to have to flex.

It's important that you wear the proper shoes to protect your Achilles tendon. There are many injuries that can be tied back to having the wrong kind of shoes. Having the wrong kind of shoes makes it only a matter of time before you sustain some kind of damage to your body tissue or muscles.

The best way to prevent injury to your muscles and joints is to make sure that you have the best walking shoes that you can afford to buy. Your shoes should be your biggest investment.

Though they're not meant to last forever, they are meant to make your walking experience comfortable. When you start a walking program, you want to make sure that you don't go all out and push yourself in a new pair of shoes.

Wear your shoes for a little while each day until you break them in so that you're comfortable in them during longer distances. Too many walkers keep their shoes for far longer than it's safe to - just because they're not aware of when the shoes should be replaced.

But there are some signs that you can check for to see if it's time for you to buy a new pair. Signs that your shoes need replacing are worn soles, uneven heels and tearing on the cushioning.

Look for cracks in the material or on the heels. Any damage or uneven places can make it easier for you to trip. The time to replace your shoes is before you actually need to.

By the time the shoes are worn down, you're at risk of injury. A good rule of thumb is the 3 or 500 rule. If you've used the shoes for 3 months and you've logged 500 miles wearing them, it's time to replace them.

Some walkers will automatically replace their shoes after 350 miles of use, but it's only necessary at that mileage if the shoe shows wear. Think of it like you would a car and making sure you get the oil changed so that the vehicle runs properly.

CHAPTER 8
Make Your Walking Program More Challenging

Beginnings are great. When you begin something new, you feel excited, energized and ready to charge ahead. But then, after awhile, it's not new, the excitement has worn off, and you don't really feel energized.

You feel stuck. Like you're just going through the motions because you know you're supposed to. When you do something for awhile, you can become accustomed to it.

You can reach a point where you can do it on autopilot - never really engaging in what you're doing. As time passes, you can also reach a certain level, known as a plateau.

When you get to this point, this means that no more changes are currently taking place. It also means that any progress you were making has now come to a stop. You've reached a point where you're no longer gaining rewards.

You won't be going backward, you simply aren't moving forward. And that's something that you always want to do - keep moving forward. This is what happens regardless of how you're trying to move more.

It happens with hard exercise, easy exercise and it happens with walking. If you're not changing up your walking program to make it more challenging, you will (at some point) reach the place where you're in a plateau.

What causes frustration with reaching this point is that you're still doing what you're supposed to do. You're making sure you get in your steps, you're being faithful to take care of your health in other ways - and yet, it feels like you're spinning your wheels.

In the beginning of a walking program, there's a payoff. You start feeling better. As you move more, you're gaining some health benefits. Your blood pressure is great.

You've gained some flexibility in your joints, some strength in your muscles. You feel more alive. You've noticed that you're losing some weight. Toning up. Your clothes fit better or you even have to buy smaller sizes.

You might feel an upswing in your moods because of walking. You enjoy breathing in the fresh air. These are all part of your reward with walking. Everyone loves a reward-based system.

You do your part and you get something in return. Then the day comes when you're doing your part and you're getting nothing in return. There's no reward just another day of walking.

What happened is that your reward got swallowed up in familiarity. Remember that familiarity is the forerunner of a plateau. Don't let your walking program become so familiar to you that you can do it on autopilot.

There's nothing wrong with wanting to see results with your walking program - with wanting to feel that sense of accomplishment or reward. Making your walking program more challenging can be a great way to avoid boredom, too.

In fact, you should review your walking goals regularly - and while you're reviewing them, you should make changes to your routine at the same time. For beginning walkers, reaching a plateau isn't something that will happen right away.

But, if you're not a beginner walker and you're ready to move up a level, then you can take steps to make your walking program more challenging. By raising the stakes, you'll get more from your program and it will be better suited to the fitness level that you've achieved.

You can start by walking briskly like you normally would - but don't keep up that pace the entire distance of your walk. Instead, keep up the brisk walk for just 5 minutes.

Then after the five minutes, walk slower for a couple of minutes. After the couple of minutes passes, go back to the 5 minutes of brisk walking until you've completed the length of time that you've become used to walking.

What this type of interval walking does is to get your heart rate elevated. It also helps you shake your body out of its routine by making it work harder in a shorter amount of time.

If you've been walking on flat surfaces, you can add a hill or incline to your journey. This elevates the amount of effort that's required from your body. But you only want to do this if you have shoes with good shock absorption.

You can challenge yourself by changing the distance that you've normally been covering. Sometimes, this can quickly shake your body out of a plateau. What you can do is instead of walking your usual 5 miles is you can push on until you go an extra mile.

But you can also do the opposite and walk a mile less than your usual 5. This throws your body out of its rut and it's a good way to shake up the routine. Remember that in order to break a plateau, all that's required is change.

You can pick a walking route that's more challenging for you to accomplish in the same amount of time. This is a change that will also work on a treadmill. All you have to do is make the incline more difficult.

Alternate your walking pace in briskness, stride and continuity. You can walk for a few minutes, then stop and do a push up or a step up. This change will help you make your walking program more challenging because your body is forced to adapt.

You can also make a walking program more challenging by pushing your pace to make sure you cover your miles in less time each time you do it. For example, if you're covering a mile in 15 minutes, push yourself to cover that same mile in 12-13 minutes.

You can challenge yourself against your own record or with a walking partner. If you use a music device while you're walking, you can make it more challenging by keeping up a brisker pace for the length of more fast paced songs than you did in the past.

Or you can switch your current playlist for an extended playlist to get more walking steps in for the day. By making your walking program more challenging as you go along, you'll avoid plateaus and the motivation to keep on going will stick with you.

Walking is a fitness activity that can be completely tailored to your preferences and needs. You can spend as much or as little on gadgets and equipment as you want. Plus, there will always be ways you can break out of a plateau with ease

BOOK EXCERPT (2015 NEW YEAR DIET SUCCESS PLAN: ELEVATE YOUR HEALTH AND HAPPINESS BY CHANGING THE WAY YOU VIEW DIETING!)

The following is an excerpt from the book: 2015 NEW YEAR DIET SUCCESS PLAN: ELEVATE YOUR HEALTH AND HAPPINESS BY CHANGING THE WAY YOU VIEW DIETING!

Learn more by checking it out on Amazon and read the first 2 chapters for free: http://amzn.com/B00RKNR8IM

BOOK EXCERPT (HOW TO CHOOSE A DIET YOU WON"T GIVE UP ON: SIMPLE WAYS TO HELP YOU ACHIEVE YOUR GOALS)

The following is an excerpt from the book: HOW TO CHOOSE A DIET YOU WON"T GIVE UP ON: SIMPLE WAYS TO HELP YOU ACHIEVE YOUR GOALS

Learn more by checking it out on Amazon and read the first 2 chapters for free: http://amzn.com/B00ROHWKXM

CONNECT WITH JESSY

Thank you so much for taking time to read this book!

If you would like to connect please check out my Facebook page

https://www.facebook.com/JessyLifeStyleChange?ref=hl

ABOUT THE AUTHOR

Jessy Colter herself struggles with weight loss. Jessy has come to the cold hard facts that dieting does not work for her. Jessy has changed her thought process to not dieting but to a life style change. Jessy wants to share information on making a life style change, which can possibly help other on their journey to their weight loss. Jessy shares her home with her three dogs which enjoys watching WWE with her. Jessy and her dog's favorite wrestler is the Undertaker. This is one of Jessy guilty pleasure. Jessy hopes that this book will help you to achieve weight loss. You can read more of Jessy books at:

http://amazon.com/author/jessycolter

ONE LAST THING

Thank you for reading this book! If you enjoyed it or found the information useful and especially if you used the information to produce results please post a short 2-3 sentence review on Amazon. I would appreciate it so much. Your support really does make a difference and I read all the reviews personally so I can get your feedback and make this book even better.

If you'd like to leave a review then all you need to do is leave it on Amazon and the link is simple to remember

Your review link here http://amzn.com/B00TXXAP46

That's it.

Thank you!